Synthetic Marijuana

Understanding Synthetic Weed and What You Need to Know

I0484170

Table Of Contents

Introduction

First off, I really want to thank you for downloading this book. This short e-book is for people who are interested in learning more about synthetic marijuana and are not sure where to start or what information to rely on. The internet today has many articles and misinformation about synthetic marijuana that confuse people who are interested in learning about this revolutionary craze and possibly interested in trying it out themselves.

In this book I am going to give you a short, concise guide for everything you need to know about synthetic marijuana. Understanding the history of these products as well as the current innovations in the marketplace are key to predicting what the future will hold. We will also go over the different health issues and what the differences and similarities are, as compared to natural marijuana.

Most importantly, we will go through the pros and cons of using synthetic marijuana so that you can understand the crucial information before taking the plunge and trying it out for yourself. Whether you plan on buying synthetic marijuana, want to know the health risks involved, or you just want to know more about why this trend has become so popular, it is important to know all the benefits and risks involved.

As a side note, I recommend that you take notes while you are reading this book. This will ensure that you get the most out of the information in here. I want you to feel that you made a purchase that was worth your money and so that you can look over the notes of this book even after you've finished reading it. The notes will help you to pinpoint exactly what you need to know and by writing things down, you will be able to recall specifics and how to handle certain situations when they arise.

Lastly, remember that everything in this book has been compiled through research, my own experiences, as well as the experiences of others, so feel free to question what you have read in this book. I encourage you to do your own research on the things that you want to look deeper into. The more you understand about synthetic marijuana, the more educated your decision-making process will be when it comes to purchasing it or being offered to try it in a social situation.

Chapter 1:

The Basics of Synthetic Marijuana

As a general rule, the government does not tolerate drugs and/or substances that can negatively affect the public's health. Due to this framework, they develop laws that prohibit or regulate drugs like methamphetamine, cocaine and marijuana (the negative effects of marijuana are still debatable). With the potential demand, some manufacturers have discovered ways to create synthetic drugs containing certain chemicals found in the natural ones without legal restrictions and consequences.

Take, for example, synthetic marijuana. Synthetic marijuana is one of those synthetic drugs that is quite popular nowadays. In fact, a 2012 statistic from the National Institute on Drug Abuse stated that 11 percent of American high school seniors used synthetic marijuana in the past year.

With the growing popularity of synthetic marijuana, a better understanding of this designer drug is essential.

What is Synthetic Marijuana?

Synthetic marijuana is a man-made drug that has similar effects to natural cannabis. This artificial drug is made in a lab where incense, herbs and other leafy materials are sprayed with liquid chemicals containing tetrahydrocannabinol (THC). Tetrahydrocannabinol (THC) is an ingredient present in the naturally-grown marijuana plants. A synthesized liquid chemical containing THC may imitate the effect of real cannabis.

Fake weed usually looks like a mixture of dried leaves from various medicinal plants. It comes with different colors, packages and branding and the public can buy these in small pockets of plastic or foil. Synthetic marijuana on the market has different flavors, ranging from chocolate to vanilla to strawberry.

What are the herbal essences found in synthetic marijuana?

The various brands of synthetic marijuana claim that they contain medicinal herbs. These herbs might include blue Egyptian water lily, dwarf skullcap, beach bean, Lion's tail, Indian warrior and Indian lotus. However, one study discovered that some synthetic marijuana products do not contain medicinal plants. In fact, a pocket-size of synthetic weed might contain nothing but lawn clippings and dried leaves sprayed with synthesized chemicals.

Composition of Synthetic Marijuana

There are many various compounds present in synthetic marijuana. HU-210, CP 47, 497 and homologues like JWH-018, JWH-073, JWH-398, are among these compounds. The cannabinoid compounds in synthetic weed acts as the cell receptors, similar to the THC found in natural marijuana.

In contrast, cannabinoid compounds in some forms of synthetic weed are stronger to THC receptors than regular marijuana. These synthesized compounds can be up to 100 times more potent than the average THC in natural weed.

How does synthetic marijuana work?

Synthetic marijuana is used in the same manner of consuming natural marijuana. It can be consumed by smoking through a pipe, bong or other device. Some users roll the synthetic weed into a joint with tobacco. There are also synthetic marijuana users who mix the drug with baked foods, like brownies, or make it into a tea.

Additionally, synthetic marijuana that is available commercially has been introduced with different names, brands and packages. It can be sold online or even at convenience stores and local gas stations.

Users of synthetic marijuana have stated that they have experienced similar effects produced by natural marijuana. They can experience altered perception, relaxation and elevated mood when smoking synthetic weed. The effects of synthetic cannabis are greater compared to natural marijuana plants because of synthesized chemicals. It can also lead to psychotic effects, ranging from hallucination to paranoia to extreme anxiety.

Why is it popular?

There are different factors for why synthetic marijuana is so popular nowadays. For one, people who smoke natural weed are turning to synthetic marijuana as a substitute. Because the state and federal law in the U.S. prohibits the use of natural cannabis, it is likely that marijuana users are purchasing artificial weed to obtain the same sensation from marijuana without legal risks and criminal consequences.

Secondly, it is popular with drivers because it cannot be detected by simple toxicology tests. This means that drivers might drive under the influence of synthetic weed without being punished by the law. It is also not detectable in most drug tests for jobs, schools, or other tested activities.

Finally, many teenagers and young adults can easily purchase synthetic weed. Unfortunately, the exposure of the young adults and teenagers to synthetic marijuana may result in health consequences that they are not yet aware of.

Chapter 2:

Synthetic Marijuana: History and Development

The Unintentional Discovery of Artificial Marijuana

Synthetic marijuana was invented by John Huffman. Huffman created the formula for synthetic weed, which composed of different chemical and herbal blends that imitated the effects of THC. Accordingly, Huffman did not intend to invent the formula for artificial weed. Due to his unintentional discovery, his initials, JWH, are used to name chemicals found in cannabinoid compounds like JWH-018 and JWH-073.

John Huffman is an organic chemistry professor at Clemson University. He began researching a class of cannabinoid compounds 25 years ago with the funding from the National Institute of Drug Abuse. He found out that cannabinoids are connected to receptors in the brain, the same with the THC of regular marijuana.

In 1995, Huffman's students manufactured 100 milligrams of JWH-018, a synthetic cannabinoid. His students tested the compound on mice and recorded their results. Huffman and his research team forgot the JWH-018, but several years later, the cannabinoid compound resurfaced as a substance for a smoking mixture that served as a substitute for natural marijuana.

Sources have claimed that Huffman was not involved in creating any synthetic marijuana being sold in the market. It added that entrepreneurs have copied Huffman's formula from his published papers.

History

Based on Psychonaut Web Mapping Research Project, "Spice", a brand of synthetic marijuana initially appeared in Europe in 2004. Spice was first introduced by a company called The Psyche Deli in the United Kingdom. Spice gained popularity in 2006, increasing the company's assets from €65,000 in 2006 to €899,000 in 2007. The brand "Spice" is also recognized in 21 countries.

Due to Spice's popularity, the other synthetic weeds introduced in 2008 were also referred to as "Spice". In fact, all herbal medicinal plants related to synthetic marijuana are dubbed as "Spice."

When artificial marijuana blends were sold in 2000, the product claimed that it may achieve similar effects of natural marijuana through a mixture of medicinal and herbal plants.

Controversy arose, however, when a 2008 laboratory analysis in Germany and elsewhere discovered something else. The analysis claimed that many of the active ingredients listed on the packet were not actually present in Spice products. The researchers also discovered large amounts of synthetic tocopherol. The study suggested that the actual plant ingredients found in synthetic weed might not be similar with what were on the labels of Spice products. It was unclear where synthetic tocopherol came from.

Different Types of Synthetic Marijuana

"Spice" or K2 are two of the most popular brands of synthetic marijuana. A wide variety of herbal blends that produce the same effects of natural cannabis are also referred to as "Spice." It is sold in different kinds of packages that go by various names such as fake weed, Skunk, Yucatan Fire, Moon Rocks, etc.

The drugs' packaging states that the products are not intended for human consumption. However, the design, marketing and labeling of Spice products allude that the products are to be inhaled or smoked as a drug. The packages also claim that it contains shredded and dried plant material sprayed with chemical additives that mimic the effect of natural marijuana.

Here is the list of other popular brand names for synthetic weed:

K2

Spice

iAroma

Voo doo doll

Diablo

Scooby Snacks

Mr. Nice Guy Jeffrey

Cloud 9

Mr. Nice Guy

Mary Joy (strong)

Hayze

Mr-Kwik-e

Peace of mind

Parade

Black Magic smoke

Atomic bomb

Spice mixtures are available in head shops, gas stations and online. Although most labels of spice products claim that it contains natural herbs sprayed with chemicals, certain analysis showed that the products contain artificial cannabinoid compounds.

Because there are certain laws implemented to prohibit the chemical compounds present in synthetic weed, manufacturers are trying to avoid legal restrictions by using different chemicals in the mixtures.

Chapter 3:

Is Fake Weed Still Legal?

Synthetic marijuana is often marketed as "legal high." It is also introduced as herbal blends or herbal incense, which are usually smoked by users.

However, there are various European countries that initially banned the synthetic cannabinoids found in synthetic marijuana. For example, since January 22nd, 2009, Germany banned the usual cannabinoid compounds of artificial weed such as CP 47, 497 and JWH-018, C6, C8 and C9 homologues.

On February 24th, 2009, France banned CP 47, 497 and its homologues, JWH-018 and HU-210.

United Kingdom, Switzerland, Russia, Poland and several countries in Asia and South America made synthetic marijuana illegal.

The United States later followed the ban after the U.S. Drug Enforcement Administration used its emergency powers to prohibit synthetic cannabinoids for a month on November 24th, 2010. Before this announcement, there were other states that created a law that prohibited and regulated synthetic weed.

The synthetic marijuana drew more controversy after an apparent suicide of an American teenager named David Mitchell Rozga on June 6th, 2010. According to sources, Rozga committed suicide by using a hunting rifle and shot himself in the head. The teen reportedly smoked K2 nearly one hour prior to the incident. Investigators believed that the young man was under the influence of a psychoactive substance at the time. Rozga's death was used as an example to help the public become aware of the dangers imposed by artificial marijuana.

After the incident, Senator Chuck Grassley of Iowa proposed a bill that would prohibit the use and distribution of the synthetic marijuana. The proposal was signed into law by the United States Congress in June of 2011.

On March 1st, 2011, the U.S. considered five cannabinoids found in fake weed- JWH-018, JWH-200, JWH-073, CP-47, 497 and cannabicyclohexanol as illegal drugs under Schedule I of the Controlled Substances Act. This meant that it was illegal to possess or use synthetic marijuana in the U.S. that contained those cannabinoid compounds. The Drug Enforcement Administration stated that the ban was aimed at preventing potential hazards posed by synthetic marijuana.

In July of 2012, President Barack Obama signed a bill called the Drug Abuse Prevention Act of 2012 into law. This law placed the artificial compounds found in synthetic weed under Schedule I of the Controlled Substance Act, making it illegal to use, possess or distribute within the United States.

Chapter 4:

Why Synthetic Weed Can Be Good For You

Studies suggest that regular marijuana is a valuable plant that helps in treating a wide range of clinical complications. Much like natural cannabis, synthetic marijuana can have a therapeutic effect. In fact, artificial cannabinoids had religious and medicinal purposes for more than 2,000 years. A newly systematic review and meta-analysis revealed the use of cannabis in treating chronic pain, such as headaches.

According to sources, there are various reasons why cannabinoids can treat a headache. First, cannabinoids can be found in areas of the brain that are involved in migraine pathophysiology. An endogenous compound called anandamide could change the pain. The presence of 5-HT1A and 5-HT2A receptors might be involved in the therapeutic effects of cannabinoids for headaches.

Secondly, migraines or headache disorders could occur from endocannabinoid deficiency, where levels of anadamide are lower. The lower levels of anadamide may then increase the activation of the trigeminal vascular system, resulting in frequent migraine attacks. However, cannabinoid receptors found in several areas of the brain might also be migraine generators.

Currently, there are a small number of published reports indicating the possible therapeutic benefits of cannabinoid drugs. These reports state that cannabinoids may aid treatment of cluster headaches, migraines, and other types of headaches. One case study revealed a patient's cluster headache attack was lessened within 5 minutes after inhaling marijuana. An alternative cannabinoid drug called dronabinol provided relief within 15 minutes as well.

In France, a survey found that 26 percent of 113 patients suffering from cluster headaches consumed cannabis to help them cope. However, it was unknown what portion of the patients used marijuana for treatment or recreational use.

Cannabinoids may be used in treating acute headaches as well. However, further studies regarding this assertion are lacking.

Synthetic marijuana helps cancer patients

In 2006, Reuters reported about a study that confirmed potential benefits of synthetic marijuana to cancer patients. According to the report, a synthetic version of the active ingredient found in marijuana is used as a legal treatment for nausea in cancer patients. The researcher also added that synthetic cannabinoids help patients experiencing symptoms like anxiety, pain and depression.

The study involved a drug called nabilone, which was sold under a brand name Cesamet. This drug was approved by the U.S. Food and Drug Administration and has been available in Canada for years. In May, the FDA approved Cesamet for cancer patients who are not responding properly to conventional anti-nausea treatments. Nabilone has cannabinoids, which is an active ingredient in natural marijuana.

The research was based upon the questionnaires answered by cancer patients. The questionnaires revealed that those patients treated with the synthetic cannabinoids experienced lesser pain compared to those who received conventional therapies. Scores for tiredness, appetite and drowsiness were stable in the Cesamet group unlike in the non-Cesamet group. With regards to the nabilone group, depression and anxiety in patients were reduced, but increased in the non-nabilone group.

The researcher added that using synthetic cannabinoids can lower the use of other drugs, which are more expensive, burdensome and may inflict more health risks to cancer patients. Additionally, this study was presented at the San Antonio Breast Cancer Symposium in the United States.

There have also been several studies conducted that show positive results from using synthetic cannabinoids to stop the spread of cancer cells:

On August 15th, 2004, the Journal of American Cancer Research reported that marijuana ingredients prohibit the spread of brain cancer in human tumor biopsies. THC may also constrain the replication and activation of gamma herpes viruses, which could increase a person's chance to develop cancer.

A research team at Madrid's Complutense University in 1998 found out that THC can selectively stimulate programmed cell death in brain tumor cells without affecting healthy cells. In 2000, the Nature Medicine journal stated that injections of synthetic cannabinoids killed malignant brain tumors in one-third of rodents used for the research.

In 1974, the Washington Post newspaper released the results of an experiment regarding marijuana's anti-tumor effects at the Medical College of Virginia. The research, which was funded by the National Institute of Health, discovered that marijuana damages the immune system. However, the study found that the THC, a psychoactive ingredient of cannabis, slowed the growth of breast cancer, lung cancer and virus-induced leukemia in laboratory rats. The methods extended the lives of the mice by more than 36 percent.

In 1975, an article called Antineoplastic Activity of Cannabinoids, which was published in the Journal of the National Cancer Institute, found another potential benefit of two cannabinoid compounds. Tetrahydrocannabinol (THC) and cannabinol (CBN), an active ingredient present in marijuana, could reduce the growth of Lewis lung adenocarcinoma. The researchers used mice that received THC and CBN for 20 consecutive days. The mice's primary tumor size was reduced after the THC and CBN treatment.

At the University of Milan in Italy, researchers stated that non-psychoactive ingredients in cannabis selectively targeted and killed malignant cells and prohibited the growth of glioma cells through aptosis.

Marijuana is a much better pain relief compared to OxyContin and Morphine. Reports have proven that cannabis can ease the pain of those people suffering from diseases like diabetes, cancer and multiple sclerosis as well.

Chapter 5:

Synthetic Marijuana And Its Negative Effects

The legal restrictions implemented by several countries, including the U.S., on synthetic marijuana products were due to its potential negative effects to human health. There have been a lot of studies conducted to analyze the components of this synthetic drug and its effect on users.

One of those studies comes from the 2012 DAWN Report of the U.S. Substance Abuse and Mental Health Services Administration. The report stated that the toxicity level which was caused by synthetic marijuana led to 11,400 cases of emergency room visits in 2012.

Synthetic pot use have led to complications like nausea, vomiting, agitation, high blood pressure and seizures.

Synthetic weed users who have been transported to Poison Control Centers exhibited various symptoms, ranging from vomiting to profuse sweating to hallucinations and rapid heart rate. K2, or Spice, can cause high blood pressure and may reduce blood supply to the heart, or worse, heart attacks. Cannabimimetics, the powerful chemicals found in synthetic marijuana pose health hazards as well.

Considering that most "Spice" products were not tested for safety and are often marketed as herbal incense that seems good for the health, some synthetic marijuana users abuse the product unintentionally.

Illnesses linked to fake weed

Synthetic marijuana use associated with kidney damage

Researchers and experts continue to warn the public about the dangers of synthetic marijuana. Nowadays, the artificial drug has been tied to many ill-fated diseases - one of these illnesses being kidney damage.

Kidney damage could turn fatal for an individual. In fact, health officials throughout the U.S. have reported that at least 16 cases of acute kidney injury involved synthetic marijuana users. Three of these incidents involved patients who were even hospitalized due to severe kidney damage.

The majority of these incidents were severe, so severe that five patients needed to undergo a dialysis. For this reason, the Centers for Disease and Control Prevention announced a warning in CDC's Morbidity and Mortality Weekly Report. Unfortunately, most victims of adverse effects related to synthetic marijuana use were young people, including teenagers.

Reports stated that young healthy individuals who smoke fake weed products can experience vomiting, abdominal or back pain and severe nausea. The kidney examination of these users showed abnormally high levels of amino acid and creatinine.

Researchers were unsure of the actual cause of kidney damage to patients who consumed synthetic weed. However, an analysis of fake weed samples smoked by patients discovered something else. The examination showed that five samples contained an ingredient called XLR-11. The XLR-11 was found in common synthetic marijuana products. The researchers suspected that this compound might have been responsible for the kidney complications.

Additionally, a report from the Substance Abuse and Mental Health Services Administration (SAMHSA) revealed that synthetic marijuana contributed to 11,400 emergency room visits in a year. Most of these patients were aged 12 to 29.

In another study, doctors from the University of Alabama discovered that designer drugs like Spice and K2 could cause serious kidney damage. These findings were the result of an examination involving four cases of acute coronary syndrome linked to synthetic cannabis use.

In this study, the researchers analyzed four men who were diagnosed with kidney damage. Each man was healthy but later hospitalized due to vomiting, nausea and abdominal pain after smoking the synthetic weed. The researchers noted that the males lived in the same town and the incidents happened within nine weeks.

Three males experienced an abnormally low volume of urine, resulting in an acute kidney injury. These men underwent a kidney biopsy, which revealed the death of cells in their kidneys. Death of cells in the kidney can be dangerous because these cells collect, secrete, reabsorb and transport urine from the body. The fourth male experienced a drop of blood flow in his kidney. While such cases can result in kidney failure, the patients regained the normal kidney functions in their bodies.

Based on this study, the doctors suggested that synthetic marijuana use could lead to acute kidney damage. They also suspected that the manufacturing methods of these designer drugs played a factor in the dangerous side effects it may pose to the users. Certain additives in synthetic marijuana can also be toxic to the kidney.

Spice linked to stroke and brain damage

Stroke and brain damage have been linked to synthetic marijuana following the tragic story of a Texas teen. Reportedly, Emily Bauer apparently consumed Spice at a party. The 16-year-old teen had been in an induced coma up until December 13th. Before she was hospitalized, Emily suffered a migraine, but woke up like a different person.

Her family said that the teenager experienced hallucinations and became violent. The emergency responders needed to restrain her before she was transported to a hospital. Twenty four hours later in the ICU, the teen was still violent and hurting herself.

Doctors put Emily in an induced coma to keep her safe. The doctors said that the teen's brain experienced an abnormal pressure, which may have explained her violent behavior and hallucinations. With this, they suggested an emergency surgery, in which doctors would drill a hole into Emily's skull in order to drain the excess fluid.

After the surgery, the doctors showed Emily's brain images. The family said that all white portions of the brain images were dead. From the look of it, Emily's family said that at least 70 percent of her brain was dead.

Emily's father learned that she bought the designer drug with a brand name called "potpourri". Unfortunately, potpourri is available at local gas stations and even convenience stores for anybody to purchase.

Emily Bauer is just one of the people who was hospitalized due to synthetic marijuana. In fact, the Substance Abuse and Mental Health Services showed that synthetic marijuana was supposedly responsible for 11,406 drug-related emergency hospital visits in 2010. Of these, children from the ages of 12 to 17 was the age-group who had the most emergency visits. Even more scary is the fact that these are crucial years for the brain to develop in these youngsters.

In a national survey conducted by the University of Michigan, one in every nine high school seniors admitted to consuming synthetic marijuana in 2011. Fake weed is the second-most popular illegal drug that these high school seniors used, followed by the much safer, natural marijuana.

While there are state laws that prohibit synthetic drugs like fake weed, the manufacturers of these synthetic drugs are doing everything they can to avoid legal restrictions. There are drug makers who slightly change the chemical ingredients of fake weed products. With this, the newly added chemical compound is not covered by the implemented law. In essence, they try to stay one step ahead of the law at all times.

Fake weed poses a higher risk of psychosis

Research presented at the American Academy of Addiction Psychiatry 22nd Annual Meeting & Symposium suggested that synthetic marijuana use poses psychotic hazards. Synthetic marijuana, although having compounds similar to natural marijuana, reportedly lacks any anti-psychotic protective agent present in regular cannabis. Due to this, people smoking fake weed are at a higher risk of suffering from psychosis.

The team of researchers began to investigate the link between psychosis to synthetic marijuana use after learning of the increasing number of psychosis cases. Their investigation discovered that these cases seemed like a substance-induced psychotic disorder.

For the research, the investigators analyzed data from Medline on studies performed from the year 2000 to 2011 and personal experiences of using Spice products together with the data from Internet resources.

The Internet sources emphasized psychotic vulnerability and addictive compounds of synthetic cannabis compared to natural marijuana. Spice users apparently experienced a long-lasting high. They also reported "hearing voices, experiencing extreme paranoia and seeing things."

Four studies conducted from 2010 to 2011 discovered that Spice users between the ages of 20 to 40 experienced confusion, anxiety and disorganization. Additionally, two of these studies reported symptoms related to psychosis with no prior psychotic disorder.

In separate research presented at the annual meeting of the American Psychiatric Association in 2011, synthetic cannabis reportedly caused long-lasting bouts of psychosis. According to sources, researchers at the Naval Medical Center in San Diego, California stated that 10 patients who were taken to a hospital due to psychosis were Spice users. Spice, the most popular form of synthetic marijuana, was also sold under the name of K2, Red X Dawn and Blaze in these cases.

In this study, the patients were ranging from ages 21 to 25. They showed symptoms ranging from paranoid delusions, thoughts of suicide and auditory and visual hallucinations. Most of the 10 patients recovered from the psychosis after five to eight days. However, some people experienced psychotic symptoms for a longer duration and recovered from it after three months.

Chapter 6:

Synthetic Weed Compared to the Real Thing

Some synthetic marijuana users think "Spice" products are much better compared to natural marijuana plants because it is supposedly legal and organic. This might seem to be true considering that synthetic marijuana manufacturers labeled synthetic marijuana as "herbal incense" consisting of different medicinal plants and certain chemicals.

However, synthetic weed has some key differences from natural marijuana and natural marijuana is becoming more accepted as safe in the public's eye. As the famous saying goes, "nobody has ever died from smoking a joint".

The cultivation process of natural marijuana is different from creating synthetic weed

Natural weed come from carefully cultivated marijuana plants while fake weed is produced from supposedly dried leaves and other scraps in a laboratory. These dried materials are sprayed with certain chemicals that mimic the effects of THC.

Manufacturers of synthetic marijuana claim their products are all natural due to medicinal plants and other ingredients. However, such claims are misleading.

Synthetic marijuana can contain anything

Generally, fake weed and natural marijuana both contain THC, a psychoactive ingredient that produces a "high" sensation. However, studies have revealed that certain "Spice" products might contain anything. Fake weed that comes in colorful packages with different flavors may have chemicals and additives that could be harmful for one's health. Artificial marijuana can be addictive unlike natural weed and this is because we do not know what the extra ingredients are in many cases.

Some people who have smoked synthetic marijuana for a long time have stated that fake weed addiction is similar to an opiate addiction. In some cases, addiction to synthetic marijuana can be physically addictive and its symptoms may include tremors, high level of heartbeat and nausea. On the other hand, natural marijuana lacks these harmful effects.

Fake weed can be up to 100 times stronger

Artificial cannabinoids can be far more powerful, depending on the chemicals used in Spice products. A report stated that the compound of synthetic marijuana is similar to DNA, and some of the chemicals containing the compound could be 1 to 800 times more powerful.

Unfortunately, fake weed manufacturers can easily change and develop the compounds to avoid legal repercussions. As the different compounds are added to Spice products, the greater the risks are to users.

Artificial marijuana is more expensive

With the constant effort of manufacturers to avoid legal restrictions of synthetic marijuana, the high price of Spice products is not a surprise. According to reports, one-gram bags of fake weed may cost $25 each.

In contrast, the street value of natural weed costs 40 percent less, for nearly $14 per gram. In addition to that, the natural high of fake weed doesn't last that long, which means that the user needs to buy more to satisfy themselves.

Synthetic weed can kill

Certain studies suggest that using synthetic marijuana as a substitute can turn fatal. In fact, there have been reports of synthetic marijuana users dying and/or experiencing life-threatening negative effects after smoking fake weed. In New York City, a 45-year-old man high on K-2, tried to surf on top of a moving subway car. Tragically, the man died shortly after his attempt.

In Texas, an 18-year-old teenager died after ingesting fake weed, which he bought at a local smoke shop. The most recent known victim of artificial cannabinoid is an 18-year-old young man named William Tucker. The young man allegedly went to a party with his friends where he stayed there until morning.

Tucker's friends woke him up the next morning around 8:30 am, so they could go to another friend's house. At the time, Tucker thought he was still drunk so he stayed and went back to sleep. Unfortunately, when his friends tried to wake him up again, Tucker was found dead. An autopsy confirmed that he died due to K2, a brand of synthetic marijuana.

Conclusion

Thank you again for downloading this book!

I hope this short e-book was able to help you learn more about synthetic marijuana, what it is made of, the different options you have, and the positive and negative effects of consuming it. Now that you have learned the important factors regarding synthetic marijuana, you can finally decide if you want to try it, or if you can inform your friends who ask you about it. Plus, a little addition to your knowledge doesn't hurt, right? It's good to know about new innovations because it keeps you in the know and up-to-date in a world where synthetic marijuana is popping up in every gas station and corner store.

Finally, if you enjoyed this book, please take the time to share your thoughts and send me a message or even post a review on Amazon. It is greatly appreciated and I try to respond to as many as possible!

Thank you and good luck in your journey!

www.ingramcontent.com/pod-product-compliance
Lightning Source LLC
Chambersburg PA
CBHW070943180526
45168CB00003B/1158